No Hogwash Allergies

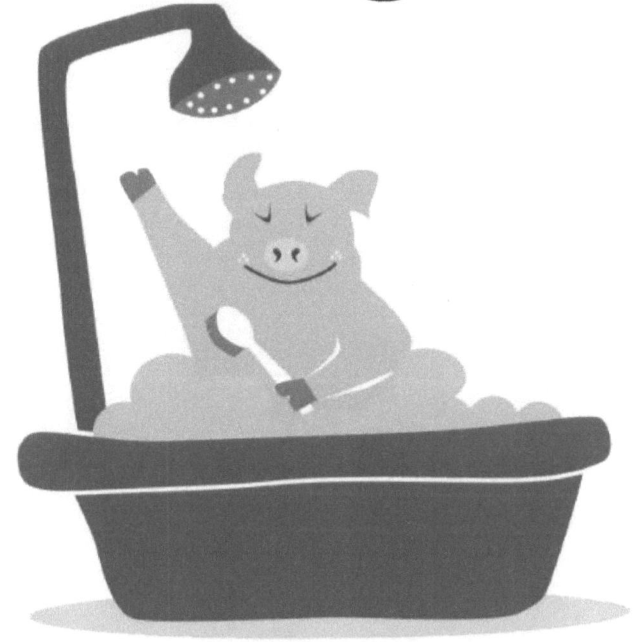

Natural Healing

By: Michael Von Irvin, MBA, BSN, RN

*It is not the strongest of the species that survives, not the most
intelligent that survives. It is the one that is the most adaptable to
change.*
—Charles Darwin

Testimonials
For Michael Von Irvin

Michael
"My pleasure to add a distinguished professional, such as
yourself, to my circle of friends. All the best to you and your
loved ones."
Father of Steve Job's Founder Of Apple Computers
John Jandali

Author • "America's #1 Marketing Wizard" •
• "The Deal Maker" • "Master Negotiator"
A lot of people are saying great things about Mike Von Irvin.

Former New York City Healthcare executive. Former VP of
AlphaCare and Director of Marketing for MLTC Consulting.
Serial Entrepreneur.

Past appearances with Geraldo Rivera, Thomas Mesereau
(Michael Jackson's Attorney), Tracy Morgan, Prince Royce,
Rafael Furcal and many other celebrities, politicians, and sports
stars.

BRANDING—My friend marketing whiz Michael Von Irvin says
branding is pointless without good Copywriting to back it up. I
think he's right.
—David Garfinkel (copywriting legend)

John Fleck
Owner
Wanted to give a shout out to Michael Von Irvin. In one day
his coaching and guidance has made a huge difference in the
direction of my business.

—Brad Szollose with Michael Von Irvin.
My second business meeting in the city was with businessman, speaker and trainer Michael Von Irvin and his wife Bella.

Some of our clients have included large healthcare plans such as AlphaCare NY - now Magellan Health. Fitango - innovative patient engagement solutions help to reduce costly readmissions and improve outcomes - NY, Special Touch Homecare LHCSA NY, ASDC, MD's, Nurse Practitioner Groups, FESCO Fire Equipment Company Birmingham/Atlanta/International, Irvin Brother's World Imports, IFPA - International Fire Protection Academy, Hood Master, Southern Fire Solutions, NAFFCO - Dubai, Exit Logic, Jessup Mfg - Chicago, MeridianRx (PBM) - Detroit, and other Healthcare Plans, Providers, Clarity, Tyco, SimplexGrinnell, FireMaster, Clinical, IT, Businesses, Marketing Related Companies, US Military Iraq.

Introduction

This book is not meant to be a masterpiece of grammar. There may be grammatical mistakes. In the spirit of No Hogwash Books, we just try to get straight to the point and to hammer these points home. We are honored that you chose this book to read and study. Some topics in this book may be covered repetitively intentionally.

REMEMBER: It is what you get out of a book that is important. This book is not meant to cover all portions of the subject. It is meant to help you. In order to learn more and grow more we also have courses designed for each subject of interest.

Thanks so much. We are very grateful to consider you a friend.

For more info visit **www.michaelvonirvin.com**
Or **www.nohogwashbooks.com**

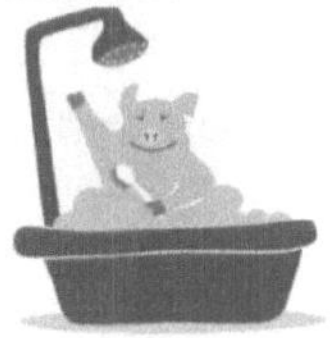

If you are going to make a real change for the better, it will not be easy at first. And know this…..there are a lot of people who are looking out for your best interest. However, there are also a lot of people who will try to control you. I had to break free of negative people and learn how to live my life to the fullest.

- *Michael Von Irvin*

Thank you for purchasing this eBook.

Sign up for my FREE eNewsletter and receive special offers, access to bonus content, and info on the latest new releases and other great eBooks from

Michael Von Irvin

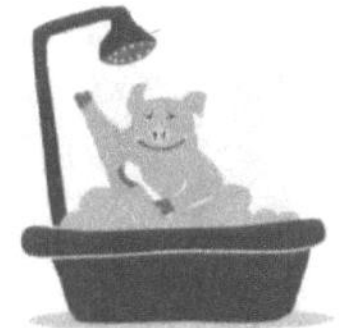

visit us online to sign up

at **www.michaelvonirvin.com**

No Hogwash Allergies

The Healthy Way to Get a Handle on Allergies

Michael Von Irvin, MBA, BSN, RN

Table of Contents

To work with Michael Von Irvin or make comments contact
help@writersprofitguide.com

Disclaimer

Nothing in this book should be construed to be medical advice or even the advice of a nutritionist or dietician. All of the comments herein are from personal experience. The author is absolved from any responsibility regarding any results from those who carry out the suggestions related in this book. Each reader is responsible for his or her own actions.

Introduction

Swollen, watery eyes, runny nose, sneezing, cough, congestion, sinus headache, fatigue, low energy…!

"It's my allergies."

"It's that time of year again."

"My allergies are driving me nuts."

"Where's my inhaler?"

"I'm gonna have to skip work – *again*."

Strange and almost mystical condition, allergies are. Most people who suffer from allergies simply accept the fact. They're allergic; end of discussion. It's something they have to live with. The problem is their numbers seem to be ever increasing.

Our grandparents may have had occasional bouts with hay fever, but none of that generation were concerned about a list of allergens as long as your arm. It would never have occurred to them.

Compare that to this day and age when more than 50 million Americans suffer from some type of allergy. (That amounts to one in every five persons. That's a lot of runny noses!) Allergies are reported to be the sixth leading cause of chronic disease in the United States.

If that were the end of the discussion it would be bad enough. Now add to this misery the time and money that such illnesses cost.

The annual cost of allergies is estimated to be nearly $14.5 billion.

Nearly 85% ($12.3 billion) is for direct costs including $1.3 billion for doctor office visits and $11 billion for medications ($7 billion prescription, $4 billion over-the-counter).

http://www.aafa.org/display.cfm?id=9&sub=30

Seven billion dollars for prescriptions; four billion for over-
the-counter medications. Notice that is billion with a "B".
Now add to these numbers the losses due to missed work and
inability to function on the job. All that money and yet in
terms of dollars spent and people suffering, the number of
suffers continues to grow. They are none the better.

In our society, we have slowly been trained to pop a pill, get a
shot, take antibiotics, and grab the inhaler – each and every
one designed to treat (or mask) symptoms. This means a
measure of relief, and yet when the next *season* rolls around
it's the same thing all over again. Sometimes worse.

Ongoing suffering is not what one would call optimum health.
This book is designed to give a deeper look at allergies – what
they are, why they exist, what perpetuates them, what causes
the symptoms to diminish. If you have been desperately
looking for answers, you will find some of them by reading
The Healthy Way to Get a Handle on Allergies.

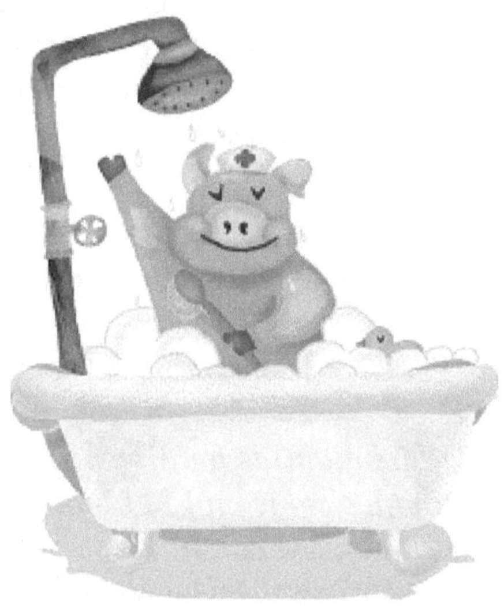

Chapter 1
What's an Allergy? What's an Allergen?

In any team sport, one of the best ways to become the winning team is to constantly study the opposing team. The coach may require that team members sit through replay after replay of a game played by the upcoming opponent. Close scrutiny of the challengers can go a long way in planning key strategies. By game time, the team is aware of how their rivals function on the field (or on the court), and are prepared for battle.

The allergy sufferer faces a formidable foe, and yet very few know what an allergy is or how, or why, it even exists. The extent of knowledge is usually something like:

"I'm allergic to cats – I have to stay away from cats."

"It's high-pollen-count time – I have to stay indoors." This might be comparable to the sports team lamenting in the locker room, "We know we're facing a monster team; we just as well get ready to lose."

Allergy sufferers have become so accustomed to losing their battle, they simply cave in. Many have spent a small fortune in over-the-counter remedies; they've been treated by specialist after specialist; they've tried this medication and that medication, but with little or no success. Quite frankly, they become disillusioned and discouraged.

If, as has been stated, the increase of allergies is a fairly recent phenomenon, and if generations past did not experience allergy suffering on today's scale, then what has changed? It's time to take a closer look and see what has happened.

What is an Allergy?

It might be interesting to note, before we dig into learning more about allergies, that farm children traditionally suffer fewer allergies than their city-bred counterparts. (One study showed a full 50 percent of children who grow up in a farm environment are less likely to develop allergies.) Statistics have proven this to be a true fact.

How can this be when one thinks of animal dander, pollen, and dust as the prime culprits in *causing* allergic reactions? Could it be because the immune systems in these children were working overtime from their earliest years?

Whatever the answer to that question, I bring in this little-known fact to demonstrate that some of our pre-supposed ideas and concepts about allergies may be out of kilter. What is the truth? What is real and valid?

The word *allergy* is derived from the Greek *allos*, which means *other*. When it was first used in the early 1900s physicians were referring to an *altered reaction* in the body's immune system. Over time, as with many terms, the meaning changed. Today allergy is a very generic term that is thrown about to apply to many problems including allergies, sensitivities and intolerances. While they are not the same things, no one seems to notice nor do they bother to clarify. This is especially true in the many general advertisements targeted to *allergy sufferers*.

Being unaware of the distinctions, many people seek medication for allergies when, in fact, they are experiencing a sensitivity to a food product.

A true allergy involves the body's immune system. A true allergy is an abnormal, adverse, physical reaction of the body to certain allergens such as dust, animal dander and pollen. (More about allergens later.) The over-active immune system sees these allergens as harmful, and thus it reacts adversely releasing body chemicals such as histamines and leukotrienes (inflammatory molecules). The immune system reacts to these outside substances that in a healthy body would be ignored.

Food sensitivities and intolerances do not involve the immune system and therein lies the main difference between the two.

Allergy specialists define allergies both by what causes them and by their various symptoms.

Causes of Allergies:

- Inhalant allergy (pollen or dust)

- Infectious allergy (symptom worsened by cold or flu)

- Insect allergy (from bite of a particular insect)

- Drug allergy (may be life-threatening)

- Physical agent allergy (adverse reaction from cold, heat, or exercise)

- Contact allergy (household chemicals, etc.)

- Food allergy (not a sensitivity – often severe)

Allergy Symptoms

- Allergic rhinitis or hay fever

- Eczema

- Hives

- Skin rashes

- Rosacea

- Anaphylactic shock (severe reaction that may be

  life-threatening)

What is Asthma?

Asthma and allergies are closely related, but are different. While an allergy is an inflammatory reaction or response to a specific substance, asthma is a chronic inflammatory lung disease that causes difficulty breathing.

The term *asthma* comes from the Greek word for *panting*. Often when an asthma sufferer is experiencing an attack they are actually gasping for air. The tubes in the lungs that deliver air (bronchi) have become inflamed. The muscles of the bronchial walls tighten and extra mucus is produced. This causes the airways to become more and more narrow shutting off air. The reason asthma is often confused with allergies is because both are often exacerbated by the same allergens – there are overlapping factors.

Asthma has become a common disease among children, and now doctors are seeing more cases of adults being diagnosed as well (adult onset asthma).

While allergy symptoms are characterized by fatigue, runny nose, sneezing, and itchy watery eyes, asthma symptoms are characterized by shortness of breath, wheezing, and coughing. Asthma sufferers often need hospitalization to get relief. Because asthma is much more life-threatening than allergies it is crucial to know the difference.

What are Allergens?

Most simply put, allergens are most anything that causes an allergic reaction. The problem is almost anything can be an allergen for someone. As has been pointed out, the immune system of an allergic person sees an allergen as harmful; therefore it reacts which then causes the allergy symptoms. Another person may experience exposure to the exact same substance and have no adverse reactions at all. (Pet dander is a good example.)

Physicians often refer to allergens as *triggers*. This is because they *trigger* (or *set off*) symptoms such as itchy watery eyes, sneezing, runny nose, congestion and so forth. While the most common allergens are such things as pollen and dust, the truth is it's possible to be allergic to most anything ranging from chlorine to perfume.

Here's a list of some of the more common allergens:

- Pollen from grass, weeds, and trees
- Proteins produced by house dust mites
- Molds
- Foods such as peanuts, tree nuts, milk, shellfish, and eggs
- Furry pets such as cats and dogs, horses, rabbits and guinea pigs
- Wasp and bee stings
- Medicines (may cause a reaction by binding to proteins in the blood, triggering the reaction)

Now that we've laid the basic groundwork of what is meant by allergies, allergic reactions, and allergens, in the next chapter we'll take look at some of the myths and truths about allergies.

Chapter 2
Conventional Treatment

The rampant onslaught of people suffering from allergies has been fairly recent. As stated in the introduction, few if any of our grandparents suffered from such a widespread list of allergies or the resulting symptoms.

As the cases have increased in number and frequencies, the medical profession and the pharmaceutical companies have raced to keep up with the problems by producing, and then prescribing, more and more *remedies, treatments,* and *medications.* The list of these treatments is now as long, or longer, than the list of allergies themselves.

Antiallergy medications have grown to become some of the most commonly prescribed drugs in the world. Add to that the fact that over-the-counter (OTC) remedies are just as popular, many of which are zealously touted in television and print ads. People desperate for relief are quick to try one after the other in the hopes that at least one or two might work. One of the problems with OTC medications is the misconception by the consumer that since a prescription is unnecessary such drugs have few, if any, side effects. Additionally they believe there's no need to inform their doctor of what they're taking. After all, what they purchase on their own is their own business. Both of the assumptions can work to the detriment of the allergic individual. The wide array of drugs available begins to cloud sound judgment.

We've already seen that the cost of the drugs is in staggering amounts of billions of dollars. They don't come cheap. Even at that, they might be worth the exorbitant cost if they actually *cured* the condition. But the best they can offer is temporary relief. Thus the allergic individual not only suffers from the condition, but also from the frustration of seeing no end to the dilemma.

Breakdown of Medications

The basic types of allergy medication fall into the following categories:

- Oral antihistamines

- Nasal Antihistamines

- Oral and Nasal Decongestants

- Nonsteroidal Nasal Sprays

- Steroidal Nasal Sprays

- Anticholinergics

- Leukotriene modifiers

Allergy Shots

In addition to the medications listed above are allergy shots (allergen immunotherapy). This is a very unpleasant treatment that involves a series of injections containing the offending allergen. As a general rule, they are given a few days apart at first, then monthly. This treatment could continue for years, and no doctor can ever predict which patient will benefit and which one will not. Because allergy shots work for only one specified allergen, that means you would need a separate shot for each thing for which you are allergic.

Side Effects

Not one of the treatments listed above are without side effects, some of which can be severe and alarming. Let's look at the first medication in the list, which is also the most common – oral antihistamines. The work of an antihistamine is to reduce the action of *histamine*. Histamine is a chemical that is released when the immune system reacts adversely to an allergen. This then leads to the release of histamine which triggers the symptoms.

Possible side effects of oral antihistamines include:

- Drowsiness

- Lightheadedness and dizziness

- Blurry vision

- Lack of ability to think clearly

- Dry mouth, nose, or throat

- Gastrointestinal upset, stomach pain, or nausea

- Increased appetite and weight gain

- Thickening of mucus

- Urinary difficulties

Next in popularity are the nasal decongestants. These may be purchased as liquids, pills, sprays, and nose drops; they can be both over-the-counter, and by prescription. The most problematic side effect is what is commonly referred to as the *rebound effect*. This means that when you stop using a decongestant, the body rebounds with even worse symptoms of nasal congestion than before. Additionally (as if the rebound effect were not bad enough) decongestants have proven to be highly addictive. Once common usage begins, it's difficult to stop.

One of the more dangerous on the list is the use of steroids. Because steroidal nasal sprays have proven to work against many of the allergy symptoms at once, they have become more and more accepted. Again, only those who suffer the misery of allergy symptoms understand the point of desperation to which one is driven just to find some measure of relief. This is why the side effects warning go mostly unheeded. However, that does not negate their reality. Here is the list of possible side effects for steroidal nasal sprays:

- Burning sensation in the nose

- Cough and bronchospasm

- Dryness in the nasal mucous membranes

- Growth suppression

- Hoarseness

- Impairment of the adrenal glands

- Increased risk of chickenpox or measles

- Insomnia

- Menstrual irregularities

- Metabolic changes (causing weight gain and increased blood glucose levels)

- Mood changes

- Nosebleeds

- Osteoporosis (a disorder in which the bones lose mass and density)

- Sore throat

- Thinning of the skin and increased bruising

- Unpleasant aftertaste

- Yeast infection

- Glaucoma

- Cataracts

- Myopathy (loss of muscle mass)

The choices of therapies for allergies are wide and highly varied. At the end of the day, all are designed to help alleviate symptoms; none are designed to solve the underlying problem (the root cause).

The best chance for allergy sufferers to live a healthy, symptom-free life is to stop, assess, research, and take a closer look at what could possibly be the root cause for the problem. In the following chapter we'll review a few theories and truths about allergies.

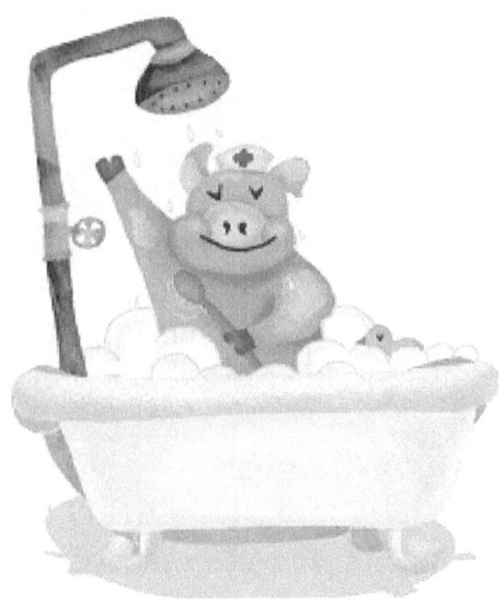

To work with Michael Von Irvin or make comments contact
help@writersprofitguide.com

Chapter 3
Myths and Theories Regarding Allergies
All in Your Head

An allergy sufferer may be told that their condition is *psychosomatic,* or in other words, all in their mind. (Those who submit that premise probably are not allergy prone.)

The suffering related to allergies is definitely real; however, the mind and emotions do play a large role in the reactions. For instance a person who is allergic to roses could experience reaction when presented with a plastic rose.

It is definitely true that emotional stress can instigate allergic reactions while relaxation techniques can lessen them. The truth is that we are totally a mind-body creature and both are closely intertwined.

Children Will Outgrow Allergies

Children are much more prone to allergies – especially food allergies – than adults. The idea that all allergies will fall by the wayside as a child's body develops is only partially true. Some individuals may move from one food allergy to another. The more common allergies that children may outgrow are dairy and eggs; the hangers-on appear to be peanuts and shellfish.

In the past it was true that children were likely to advance past the food allergies of their younger years; but today statistics are showing it's taking a much longer period of time. Meanwhile, great wisdom is required of parents to deal with these issues.

Life-Threatening or Not?

In extreme cases, allergies can definitely be life threatening. If an individual has a severe sensitivity to a certain substance it can create what is known as anaphylactic shock. When this happens the blood pressure lowers, the tongue and throat swells, the airways to the lungs are constricted and breathing becomes difficult. Immediate medical attention is required. The trigger could be a food or drug, or it could be an insect bite or sting.

One lady reported that while in a restaurant, she attempted to explain to the waitperson of her intolerance to gluten. The waitperson shot back the comment, "Well, it's not going to kill you, is it?" She had to wonder if it had to result in death before she was taken seriously.

Those with a history of such reactions know to carry a pre-loaded syringe of epinephrine (EpiPen). Epinephrine is a synthetically-produced form of the hormone adrenaline which works to reverse the effects.

Allergic to Pet Fur?

Those who suffer from allergies from furry pets know what a problem this can be. Simply visiting the home of a friend who has cats or dogs can set off the unpleasant symptoms. However, it's not the fur that is the culprit, rather it's the dander which are microscopic flakes of skin that become airborne.

While it's nice to think there are nonallergenic breeds of dogs, it's a fallacy, since all cats and dogs have skin. Short-hair or long-hair, those that shed and those that do not – there is no distinction when it comes to allergies.

Protection from Poison Ivy – Gloves and Heavy Clothing?

Wearing protective clothing and gloves may make one feel safer when taking a walk through the woods, or working around poison ivy, but it's an illusion. The truth is the oily resin (urushiol) that causes the allergic reaction can cling to clothing, the fur of a dog or cat, and even garden tools.

It's still wise to wear as much covering as possible – it will serve as the frontline prevention. However, if when removing the clothing your skin comes in contact with the resin, it can still become a problem.

Keep in mind that urushiol is tenacious in that it will remain on items such as unwashed garden tools for a long period of time. Whatever has come in contact with the plants should be thoroughly washed. (Pets included.)

Got Milk Allergies?

When adults experience adversely reactions to milk, such as cramps, gas, and diarrhea, they often mistakenly think they are allergic to milk (or dairy products). In truth, it's a condition known as lactose intolerance. This means the body suffers from a lack of the enzyme lactase which is necessary to break down lactose (the sugar in milk or dairy products). Unlike a real food allergy the lactose intolerance does not involve the immune system.

Move to the Southwest for Allergy Relief

It would be nice to think there is a "safe haven" for allergy sufferers, but alas, it is not to be. It's true that desert areas are free of maple trees and ragweed; however, there's an abundance of pollen-producing plants such as sagebrush and cottonwood, ash, and olive trees.

If you are already allergy-prone, once you move you may simply experience a fresh new set of allergies to local plants. So don't pack your bags just yet.

This chapter has touched on only a few of the myths and theories that abound regarding allergies. As can be seen allergies of all sorts and varieties are indeed serious – some even life threatening. They make life miserable for millions of sufferers and cost time and money and are a detriment to living a full healthy life.

Now that we've laid the groundwork, in the next chapter we will take a big step toward looking past the misery-causing symptoms. Let's take a look at what's going on behind the scenes.

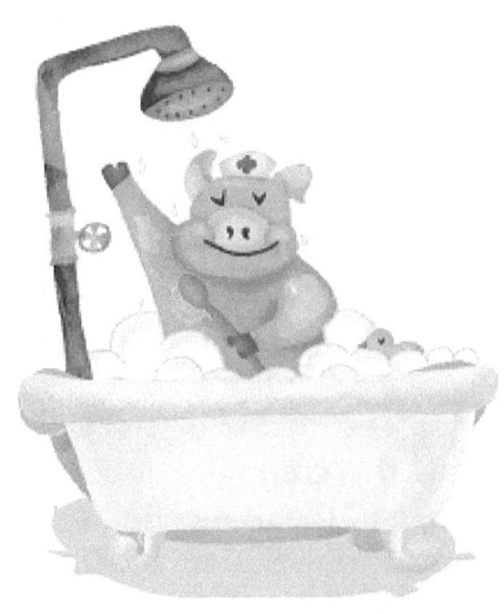

To work with Michael Von Irvin or make comments contact
help@writersprofitguide.com

Chapter 4
What Has Changed?

If indeed it's true that the allergy epidemic has developed fairly recently, it would be logical to look back over a span of time and ask, *what has changed*. Let's take a brief overview and see what we can uncover.

Time Spent Out of Doors

Talk to any senior citizen about his or her childhood, and you will most likely hear stories of running through the woods, climbing trees, playing in the creek, swimming in the pond, bicycling through all the streets of the neighborhood, or playing whatever-season ballgame in the vacant lot on the corner. School recess time was always spent playing outside, autumn, winter and spring. Bottom line, children spent the highest percentage of their time out of doors. For the most part this out-of-doors playtime consisted of unstructured, stress-free, activities in which imagination and creativity had full reign.

The scenario has changed over the past couple of generations. Children no longer play outside as much – the highest percentage of their time is spent in the house (usually in their room), or in a school building.

Not only has this resulted in a less-healthy generation, but also a generation with a complete disconnect with nature. Appreciation of nature and the things that exist in nature is stilted, and often non-existent. **Sedentary Lifestyle**

As pointed out above, being out of doors could be interpreted as *active* and *moving*. Looking back a few generations ago, by necessity people walked to where they were going. Walking several miles to get to town, or to get to school, was not considered uncommon; it was how things were.

Cars and readily-available public transportation changed that, as did the entrance of television into our culture. The evolution of computers and various hand-held technological devices have added to the condition.

Sitting became the norm whether at home, at work, or on the way. The term *couch potato* came into being for good reason. Now if one were to take a walk, it might simply be an evening stroll after dinner rather than purposeful walking to get to a destination.

While the term of couch potato came into being in the 1970s, it became even more apropos in the 1980s with the introduction of the remote control. Now it wasn't even necessary to get up off the couch to change channels on the family television. Obviously, there's a humorous side to this condition of the present generation, but the dangers and health problems cannot be ignored.

Stress, Tension, Fatigue

We live in an extremely fast-paced world compared to that of our grandparents. We might envision them sitting in their living room, or out on the front porch on a summer evening. They're listening to the music on the radio and rocking in the rocking chair or swinging in the porch swing. Conversation is slow and easy and no one is in a hurry to go anywhere.

Compare that to the pace at which we live today where a day when we are *not* hurrying to get somewhere is rare. Getting to work, attending meetings, catching appointments, plus school and sports events for the kids. It's a mad rush on a daily, and hourly, basis.

Stress builds not only from the pace at which we live but also from crises such as illness, divorce, dysfunctional relationships, an angry boss, a job we hate, and so on.

Add to this the fact that every calamity in the world is brought into our living rooms via the nightly news. If you don't have enough to worry about in your own life, just watch the news and all the problems of the world are added to the mix.

This isn't to say our forebears did not have stress. They certainly did; however, it's safe to say it was nowhere near the scale at which we experience in today's world. Ongoing, unremitting stress leads to many other physical problems (other than allergies) such as constant tension and chronic fatigue syndrome.

The Food We Eat

Of all that has been listed so far, the most drastic change in the past couple of generations has been the food that we eat. Our grandparents – even the city dwellers, enjoyed freshly-grown produce from their own gardens. The meat they ate was either the livestock they raised, or their neighbor had raised. They knew where it came from. This plus the wild game such as rabbit, squirrel, venison, and fowl that was hunted to put food on the dinner table.

Then came the evolution of canned goods sitting on the grocery store shelves and boxes of mixes and cereals decked out in attractive packages. Meat that was butchered and processed in a factory neatly lined the meat coolers in the supermarkets. The busier people's lives became, the more they turned to easy-to-fix (quick-to-fix) foods – dinners that came right out of a brightly foil-wrapped package.

Processed foods (as they are now known) were an instant gold mine for the food industry. The problems that needed solving were 1) how to make manufactured food attractive (and smell good), and 2) how to make sure they would have enough preservatives to sustain a long shelf life. These were solved and they were home free.

Slowly, over time, many food items have been transformed into substances that have little or no nutritional value, and yet people eat them thinking they are *feeding* their body.

In the name of convenience, processed food give the consumer what they want – quick, cheap food with the flavor they crave (usually sweet or salty). At the current time, the processed food industry is one of the largest manufacturing sectors in the United States.

Unlike our grandparents who went to the back yard garden and picked a few tomatoes and pulled up a few carrots for supper, when we purchase processed foods we have no idea what they contain. Nor if there is any nutritional value. Nor do we know how many, nor what types, additives, preservatives, dyes, and other various chemicals may have been added.

Water – Or Lack Thereof

Another slow and subtle change in our lifestyle has been the cessation of drinking water. In times past when a person was thirsty it meant they wanted (and needed) a drink of water. That was a given. Perhaps lemonade or tea was served with a meal, but for the most part everyone drank water.

Not so in this era. Water is often the last thing on the list when a person wants to quench their thirst. High on the list, obviously, is soda pop. The amount of sugar, caffeine and other additives in soda pop is enormous. The food value is non-existent. Next on the list might be coffee. For those who live in the south, it might be sweet tea. Add to that bottle juices and it's easy to see that water lacks a strong vote.

The sad fact is that most people fail to understand the body's basic need for water. Plain water. It's a fallacy to believe that just because a glass of iced tea contains water it's sufficient to supply what the body needs. Because our bodies are made up of 50% to 70% water, many of the organs (brain included) must have water to function properly.

Toxins in the body are allowed to build up due to the lack of *flushing* that happens when sufficient amounts of water are consumed on a daily basis. Such toxins are highly disease-related.

Toxins

Speaking of toxins, the last in this list of things that have drastically changed over the past generation is the increase in the amounts of toxins in our environment. This is in the air we breathe, in waterways, the soil and in our homes and offices. Toxins range from industrial chemicals to common household cleansers.

While it is impossible to ever totally get away from this chemical soup, it is possible to 1) eliminate many by cleaning up our personal environment, and 2) building up our immune system to enable our bodies to have a fighting chance to combat these.

As you have read through this brief overview of changes in our world, you may be wondering what this has to do with allergies. That question will be answered in the next chapter and we begin to search for the root cause of allergic reactions.

Chapter 5
The Search for the Root Cause
Body Designed to Heal Itself

Have you ever gotten a bad scratch or laceration? At the outset, it looks raw and ugly. You may apply a medicinal ointment, but for the most part, other than keeping it clean, you leave it alone. In a few days it has scabbed over. At some point that scab may fall off. A couple weeks later you forget you ever had the laceration. Only a small mark is visible to remind you that you once had a bad scratch.

What has happened here? You have just witnessed a minor miracle. You have just seen proof that the human body is designed to ultimately heal itself. This true not only on the surface of your body but hidden deep inside.

When someone has a broken bone, the doctor may set the bone, and may put the limb in a cast, but that doctor has nothing whatsoever to do with that bone knitting itself back together. It happens because the body is designed to heal itself.

Our bodies are complex machines that are intricately designed. Within itself it has a lubrication system, an intelligence system, a cooling and warming system, and the list goes on. It also has a healing system known as the immune system. The immune system is responsible for the healing of the cut mentioned above.

While you can see a cut healing, other parts – the internal parts – of your body are being healed every day through an amazingly complicated process. The vital organs as well as the systems are constantly waging an unseen war against unwanted invaders.

At the first sign of any internal inflammation, for instance, immediately a warning signal is sent. *The defenses have been breached and a destructive process is underway.* The immune system heeds the warning and sends in its first line of defense – the white blood cells. The white blood cells now mobilize to remove the invaders. In addition, there is an entire assault crew of chemicals to aid in the warfare. When the battle is won the work is still not completed. Now the body sends in the *anti-inflammatory* substances – which are manufactured from cells and absorbed from foods (healthy foods that is). You're on your way to work; you're fixing supper; you're helping the kids with their homework; you're watching your favorite television program. You have not one thought of your immune system as to whether or not it's working properly or not. Nevertheless, it is always on alert; always functioning. Or at least *attempting* to function. The trouble is, we humans are not always cooperating.

Anatomy of an Illness

Many years ago journalist and author, Norman Cousins, was diagnosed with an incurable disease. Rather than accepting that pronouncement of death, he undertook to chart his own recovery plan. All with the approval and cooperation of his doctor. He did recover and later wrote about his experience in his now-famous book, *Anatomy of an Illness* (1979).

Cousins went on to do extensive research in the field of the immune system, and in the mind-body connection of illness and healing. When he embarked upon this journey, he was dismayed to search through medical school textbooks – literally scores of them – and found *no teaching* on the immune system. How could this be possible when, as he well knew, the body's immune system is the first line of defense when something goes awry in the body?

Over-Active Immune System

So now let's tie this together with our main topic – allergies. In Chapter 1, we learned that allergies are absolutely *something going awry* in the body. Additionally allergies have everything to do with the body's immune system. Allergies, basically, are the result of an over-active immune system. In other words, an immune system that is not functioning as it was designed to function. This fact was clearly stated in Chapter 1:

> *A true allergy involves the body's immune system. A true allergy is an abnormal, adverse, physical reaction of the body to certain allergens such as dust, animal dander and pollen. The over-active immune system sees these allergens as harmful, and thus it reacts adversely releasing body chemicals such as histamines and leukotrienes (inflammatory molecules). The immune system reacts to these outside substances, that in a healthy body would be ignored.*

If this is true – and it is – then it would only make sense that the root cause of allergies is inextricably tied to the immune system. It would further make sense for an allergy sufferer to learn everything possible about the immune system – how it works, how it is supported and how it is hindered. How might an individual best cooperate with the system that is already in place?

Time to Take Control

In this *information age* many people, who are discouraged with a medical world that treats only symptoms, are getting serious about taking control of their own health and healthcare. Norman Cousins was one of the forerunners in this, but there are now thousands, if not tens of thousands, of others. People are discouraged and weary at being glanced at by a physician and then handed another prescription simply because the previous medication is not working.

This is not meant in any way to disparage medical doctors. They are squeezed into tight places by insurance demands and demands of large clinics and heavy schedules. As has been mentioned few of them are taught in medical school about health and wellness (the immune system), rather they spend years studying illnesses, diseases, and medications. Sad but true.

Taking control of your own health will mean taking responsibility. It may mean lifestyle changes; it may mean mindset changes. No one can ever force you to make crucial lifestyle changes. It's your choice. It comes down to a simple question – do you want to be well?

Now that we know the root cause of allergies predominately stems from the body's immune system, it's time to learn more about this amazing system.

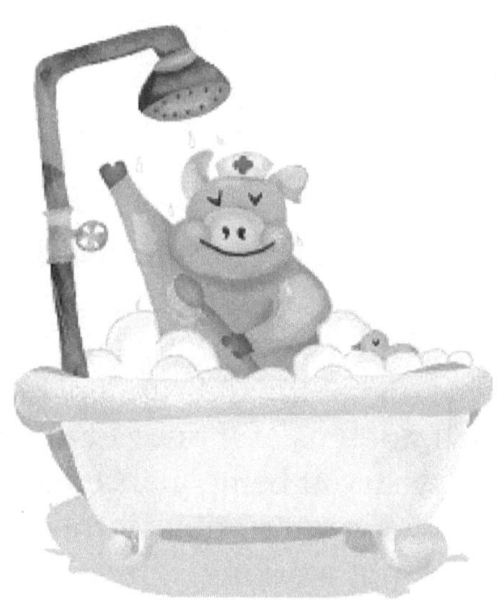

Chapter 6
Immune System Destruction

Would You Destroy Your New Car

If you were the owner of a fine new car, one that you had wanted for many years, would you purposely set about to destroy the cooling system? How about the lubricating system? The brake system? The exhaust system? Perhaps the fuel system? Would it ever occur to you that any part of the workings of this new car was expendable? Which one would you prefer to do without?

This seems such a silly question, and yet every day, in a hundred different ways, people are destroying their immune system. This is the very system within the body that is designed to fight off disease and illnesses, and as mentioned in the previous chapter, heals bodily wounds. The immune system is one of the more crucial systems, and most people haven't a clue how it works.

If your car were destroyed it's possible to purchase a new one. A body that is ravaged by illness and disease cannot be replaced. We need to learn to respect our bodies and treat them at least as responsibility as we would a car.

How the Immune System Works

The more you know how the immune system works, the better able you will be to support it. Your immune system is made up of special cells, proteins, tissues, and organs. These work as a team to defend you from germs and microorganisms every day. When operating at peak performance this system does a great job of keeping you healthy. However, if the immune system is compromised, it can lead to a wide variety of health problems.

The system operates through several steps that we call the immune response. This is when the system cooperates, works together, and attacks organisms and substances that might cause illness and disease.

The main players in the system are white blood cells (or leukocytes), which are produced in the bone marrow, but can be found in many parts of the body – including the blood and lymphatic system. The two different types of leukocytes are:

- Phagocytes: Cells that chew up invading organisms

- Lymphocytes: Cells that allow the body to remember and recognize previous invaders and help the body destroy them.

This is a simple description of the immune system which is sufficient for the subject matter of this book. In reality, of course, the workings of this system are highly intricate and would require an entire book to fully describe.

How is the human immune system damaged? Many of the ways this system is compromised can be traced directly back to the changes pointed out in Chapter 4. One of the biggest culprits is lack of exercise – the sedentary lifestyle.

Lack of Exercise

Most everyone knows the sluggish feeling that comes from sitting around for long periods of time. What is not as obvious is that the immune system is also growing sluggish. Low levels of exercise sends the message to the body that the leukocytes are not needed thus the levels begin to drop.

An indirect result of the sedentary lifestyle is the fact that sleep quality is compromised. Lack of proper rest also weakens the immune system.

Yet another indirect result of lack of exercise is the greater chance of being overweight. When the body contains a high number of fat cells, this in turn triggers the release of pro-inflammatory chemicals in the body. This will result in chronic inflammation. When the inflammation is ongoing, healthy tissues get damaged. Inflammation is one of the main symptoms of allergies.

Sugar Intake

Changes in eating habits was discussed in Chapter 4 when it was pointed out how we ingest substances in today's society that have absolutely no nutritional value. Sugar would have to be at the top of the list when it comes to the danger posed to the human body.

Gallons of soda pop, tons of candy bars – and don't forget all the truckloads of donuts and sweet desserts – are consumed on a daily basis, and yet few consumers are alarmed about it. Even these alone would present a frightening picture, but the truth is nearly every processed product on the grocery shelves contains added sugar. Those products range from catsup to salad dressing to a can of green beans. One would be hard pressed these days to find a processed food item that did not have sugar added in some form or other.

In the United States a century ago (1887-1890), an individual ingested an average of about five pounds of sugar per year. Five pounds. Any guesses what that average is today?

Today, an individual's annual intake of sugar has spiked to a mind-boggling *135 pounds*. We eat over one hundred pounds of a substance that has no nutritional value, and yet it holds a great capacity to do harm to our bodies.

One of the most serious consequences of too much sugar is that it works to suppress the immune system. Eating or drinking 100 grams (8 tablespoons) of sugar – the equivalent a couple of 12-ounce cans of soda pop – can reduce the ability of white blood cells to kill germs by 40 percent.

Processed Foods

In a similar manner processed foods offer little or no nutrition for the sustenance of the systems of the body, hence their ability to operate at top form is compromised. The increased prevalence of *junk foods* drives people to eat for taste and pleasure rather than for optimum health. Even those who know this or that product is bad for them, continue to eat it simply because it has become an ingrained habit. There's a big difference between eating just to satisfy hunger and eating for optimum health.

The term *processed foods* refers to raw food such as grains or meats that have been formed into new, more convenient and marketable food products. Processed foods make the food industries a great deal of money – at the cost of compromising the health of all who consume them on a regular basis.

Not only have nutrients been removed from processed foods, but highly dangerous chemicals have been added. Over 15,000 toxic chemicals are allowed by the Food and Drug Administration to be added to processed foods without ever showing up on the labels.

Wisdom regarding healthy eating seems to have been lost – replaced by strong influence from advertisers and marketers. This means foods that were once of value to the body have been refined, stripped of nutrients, lacking vitamins, and full of chemical additives and preservatives, thus our bodies can barely digest them, let alone assimilate them. And yet we continue to base our diets around them. As a result the immune system is progressively weakened.

Water

Lack of sufficient hydration plays a huge part in weakening the body's immune system. The problem is few people even know when they are genuinely *thirsty*, due to the sweetened caffeinated drinks that are constantly consumed. Since the thirst, the need for water, is masked most people are severely dehydrated and have no awareness.

High Stress Levels

While some stress is normal in any life, it's when increased stress is prevalent on a daily basis that health problems occur. As with the other conditions listed above, stress also works to lower the immune system's ability to resist invader germs and bacteria. People wonder why right in the middle of an important event, such as a wedding or holiday, they come down with a cold or flu. It's because the immune system was compromised by the increased stress.

Stress can shut down the digestive system which means no matter how well you eat, your body is deriving little nutrition from that food. It also means that poorly digested food is building up in the body giving off unwanted toxins. (More about toxins next.)

The fact that most people reach for the quick fix when stressed – coffee, tobacco, alcohol, drugs – further exacerbates the problem. Again because they deal with the symptoms and not the cause of the problem and as a result the immune system suffers.

High Level of Toxicity

Your liver is your primary toxin processor. For instance, if you inhale or ingest something toxic, the toxins enter your circulation and head directly to your liver. The overworked, run-down liver cannot perform this job as needed. This means toxic levels rise which then causes significant stress on the vital organs such as heart, brain, and kidneys. The lymph are now congested because the blood is unable to tolerate any more toxins coming in that your liver cannot get rid of. As mentioned toxins can result from a buildup of poorly digested foods, in addition to all of chemicals we breathe, touch, and ingest. The more toxins present in the body, the less effective the liver will be in its *cleansing processes*.

All of the areas mentioned in this chapter can help you to see more clearly what all is involved in the immune system. Back to the car example, you should no more purposely damage your immune system than you would purposely damage the brake system on your new car.

In the next chapter we'll take a different approach, discussing what you can do to keep your immune system in tip top shape. Are you ready to get serious about getting a handle on your allergies?

Chapter 7
Immune System Construction

I trust it has become abundantly clear by now that getting a handle on your allergies is not an overnight quick fix. It's not in a pill or a potion or a nasal spray. It involves discipline and commitment. It involves your will. It involves your determination to get healthy.

In this chapter we'll look at a number of very simple ways in which you can begin to support, build up, and heal your immune system. The best part is that these steps are not complicated, nor are they expensive.

By concentrating on the immune system, this in no way means that a weak immune system is the *only* cause of allergic reactions. However, it can be safely said that this is a huge factor and if it were to be remedied, in most cases, many symptoms would simply dissipate.

Exercise = Oxygen

Exercise has gotten a bad rap in today's society in that it is mainly relegated to the realm of weight loss – and Americans are obsessed with weight gain and loss. Those who want to lose weight get serious about exercise; those who aren't don't. This is a tragedy because exercise is a hundred times more connected to good health than with weight loss.

One of the most powerful benefits of aerobic exercise is how it results in deep breathing and thereby strengthening the lungs and introduces oxygen to the body.

Of all the forms of nourishment that are necessary for life, air is at the top of the list. On average an adult can consume about 2 pounds of solid food in a day, 4 pounds of liquid and nearly 18 pounds of air! You can live several weeks with no food; you can live several days with no water; but you can last no more than a few minutes with no air.

Most of us breathe and never give it a second thought. And yet it is our very breath that gives us the oxygen so necessary for life. Each and every cell in your body relies on oxygen for its very existence. Lack of oxygen results from shallow breathing; and shallow breathing happens when the body is inactive. Without proper exercise the cells begin to suffocate; oxygen reserves are not maximized and the energy supply is depleted.

Without the proper amount of oxygen, unhealthy or weak cells – due to improper metabolism – lose their natural immunity. Now the body is susceptible to viruses and opens the door to all kinds of serious health problems. Including allergies.

One of the first and easiest ways to support the immune system is with regular exercise. This doesn't mean you have to join a spa or gym – unless that's your preference. Find something you like to do whether it's biking, swimming, jogging, or even taking a brisk walk. Be creative and get your body moving. As you begin to exercise and begin breathing deeply, the lungs are being strengthened and more oxygen is being distributed to all the cells of the body.

You need at least 90 minutes a week of movement that raises your heart rate to 70% of its maximum capacity. (This can be 30 minutes three times a week.) If you haven't been exercising previously, start small and work up. Once you are up to 90 minutes a week, you will experience a noticeable difference in your energy levels. What you cannot see is how on the cellular level, each one of your cells is being revived with their fresh dose of life-giving oxygen.

Additional Benefits of Exercise

If the extra supply of oxygen gained from exercise were the only benefit, it would be sufficient; however, there are many others.

- **Weight Loss** Regular exercise burns calories. It's as simple as that. In addition to shedding pounds, exercise helps tone all the muscles of the body.

- **Elevates the Mood** Regular exercise stimulates the brain chemicals that help to elevate your mood and brings on a relaxed feeling. The more you get into a regular exercise routine the better you will feel about yourself. It boosts your confidence and improves self esteem.

- **Added Energy** Exercise helps your cardiovascular system work more efficiently which in turn gives you added energy.

- **Sleep Aid** Regular exercise not only helps you fall asleep quicker, it helps you to sleep more deeply.

- **Bone and Muscle Health** Regular exercise helps build and maintain healthy bones, muscles, and joints.

To work with Michael Von Irvin or make comments contact help@writersprofitguide.com

- **Balance** Regular exercise improves a sense of balance

  which prevents falling.

Deep Breathing = Oxygen

Yet another way to up oxygen levels – a way that is inexpensive, easy, and can be done almost anytime and anywhere – is deep breathing. Most people breathe from the top part of their lungs, known as shallow breathing.
In order to intake the maximum amount of oxygen, and in order to clean out the lungs and make the maximum air exchange, a person must breathe deeply. We want to expel as much carbon dioxide as possible and take in as much oxygen as we can. This can come only from learning to deep breathe.

The first step in deep breathing is to become aware. The breathing that you have taken for granted most of your life will now come to the forefront of consciousness. Take notice when you are shallow breathing. Then stop and begin to pull in deep breaths that allow you to breathe to the very lowest part of your lungs. Shallow breathing means old air is not exchanged for new fresh air. Here are steps that will get you started. Once you create your own habit of deep-breathing routines you will never want to stop. It clears your head and calms your nerves.
If you are a beginner at this the best position is sitting with your back straight. After you become accustomed to the routine you can deep-breathe no matter what you're doing and no matter where you're located.

- The tip of your tongue will be placed against the

  ridge behind your upper front teeth and kept there

  throughout the exercise.

- Now exhale through the open mouth while making a whoosh sound.

- Inhale through the nose with a count to four.

- Hold that breath and count to seven.

- Exhale again through the open mouth counting to eight. Again with the whoosh sound.

- This is one full deep-breath cycle. Inhale again, and repeat the entire cycle for at least three times.

Oxygen is a prime immune builder. Make exercise and deep breathing a priority in your daily lifestyle and get ready for awesome results.

Sugar

Another inexpensive way to support and aid your immune system is to slowly wean your taste buds off of sugar. A word of wisdom on this point: when making any dietary changes, take it slow and easy. Begin by eliminating one item at a time, and try to substitute with a healthier choice. If you get brash and try to go cold turkey, it's reminiscent of a crash diet and in a couple weeks you'll be right back where you started. Instead, make lifestyle changes that will last a lifetime.

An example of such a change: At ten every morning, Craig leaves his desk at work, heads to the break room and grabs a sweet roll and a cup of coffee. But now he wants to change that. In his goal to cut down on sugar intake, he begins keeping a stash of trail mix at his desk. Instead of going to the break room, he steps outside into the fresh air, takes a quick walk and snacks on the trail mix. In changing his behavior as well as his eating, the body and mind are being redirected; old habit patterns are broken.

One of the biggest culprits of sugar intake is soft drinks. The addiction to soft drinks is rampant in our nation and it's not all that easy to break free. It's the sugar plus the caffeine that is addictive. Again, be creative with ways to substitute.

If you have a habit of buying a large soft drink every time you go to the convenience store, simply stop going to the convenience store. Don't bring sodas into your home. When eating out, order water instead. Step by step you can get free.

As much as possible, avoid products that say *sugar-free*. Most of these are laden with harmful chemical sugar substitutes. The point in aiding your immune system is to seek out healthy alternatives. Sugar substitutes do not qualify. Try using natural sweeteners such as honey, stevia, agave nectar, blackstrap molasses, and barley malt syrup.

As with the exercise, by eliminating excessive sugar intake soon you will notice an increase in your energy levels. Every vital organ will begin to function as it was designed to function.

Processed Foods

The problems with processed foods were pointed out in Chapter 6, how raw foods are stripped of nutrition and then laden with harmful chemicals. The more processed foods that are consumed the less fuel the body has to work with. This would be like plugging the fuel lines in your car. Efficiency is compromised. We eat processed foods because they are quick, easy, and they taste good. To truly get serious about increasing your immune system to diminish the allergy symptoms it will require a well-laid-out strategy.

Take inventory of your refrigerator, pantry, and cupboards. What packaged products can be substituted with healthier choices? Call a family meeting and discuss the alternatives. Get everyone in on the act; let it be a cooperative effort. Little by little begin to switch out the empty-calorie, heavily-sugared items and replace with healthy foods with substance.

Begin to think about food – real genuine food – that is in a state as close to the original design as possible. This means fresh fruits and vegetables. Learn to shop the perimeter of the grocery store. It's in the center aisles where all the packaged foods are found. Every time you are tempted to slip back into grabbing a quick-to-fix package, stop and ask yourself what can be substituted.

Perhaps you might add one serving of fresh fruits and vegetables to at least three meals in one week. Instead of opening a can of green beans, buy fresh green beans in the produce section and steam them.
Make a list of the major junk-food culprits in your life and remove one a week. Always make sure there is a healthy substitute. Remember this is a strategy. Slowly cut back on the indulgences – but always leave one or two so your subconscious will be fooled into thinking there has been no change at all. This will help stave off cravings.

To work with Michael Von Irvin or make comments contact
help@writersprofitguide.com

Read health and wellness books and research healthy recipes. Instead of thinking of a package, think of how you can fix a meal in the crockpot. You get the idea.

All the systems in your body recognize a carrot. They absolutely do not recognize a helping of Doritos. Or a Milky Way bar. Or a can of soda pop. These empty calories do nothing but add stress to the systems.

This is a process of learning to respect your body and appreciating the way in which it functions.

Water

Most people are thirsty and don't know it. Sad but true. Why is that so? It's because we get so used to not drinking water our bodies adjust by simply turning off the thirst mechanism. By the time actually sense that you're thirsty, you may already be mildly dehydrated.

A dehydrated body produces more histamine – this is the very thing an allergic person is trying to avoid. Dehydration also may account for the allergy symptoms of runny nose and watery eyes.

As it has been pointed out, every organ in the body needs water – and this includes the respiratory system which is so crucial in the war against allergies. Water regulates body temperature, cushions joints, protects organs and tissues, and helps to carry nutrients to every cell in the body.

The heart, blood, and kidneys operate as a fully-functioning filtering machine. This unit, as it cleanses and purifies, works to remove all toxic waste and removes harmful substances that get into our bodies. Most of the liquids we consume work to stress this system rather than support. Only water will do the job effectively.

As with weaning off of sugar and processed foods, apply the same strategy to the drinks that you consume. Little by little begin to substitute water for the coffee, soda pop, sweetened juices, and sweet tea that you habitually drink. Drink filtered water as opposed to tap water. Try squeezing fresh lemon in a glass of water for an extra added zing.

Drinking six to eight glasses of water a day will help to flush the toxins from your body. It's these toxins that weaken your immune system and trigger allergic reactions.

De-Stress

Ongoing high levels of stress work against the immune system. As stress has increased in our society, so have our methods of alleviating stress. We look for quick relief in pills, alcohol, caffeine, and tobacco among other things. This is counterproductive as most of what is listed here simply exacerbates the stress and never touches the core problem. Natural stress relievers are readily available and simple to adopt into your lifestyle. Determine that stress will no longer rob you of optimum health.

Several of the immune-system-builders already listed in this chapter are also stress relievers. Exercise is a stress reliever, as is deep breathing. Other methods you might want to try are:

- Yoga

- Massage

- Visualization and guided imagery

- Biofeedback

- Meditation

- Hypnotherapy

Using natural means of relaxation means allowing the body to do as the body is designed to do – heal itself. If you have been on antidepressants and tranquilizers, you may be able to slowly wean off of these drugs as your body becomes more and more healthy.

As you begin to adopt healthy lifestyle changes you will find that things in your life that once caused tension and stress, no longer bother you. This is because your body is functioning at a peak performance that before was lacking.

Toxins

If, as we have already ascertained, toxins are everywhere and in everything, how is it possible to win in the battle against such an onslaught? The answer is to strengthen the immune system so it will do most of the work for you.

As you change your eating habits, you will be amazed at how many toxins you are now avoiding. Many foods and herbs when ingested become detox agents for your digestive system. Foods such as:

- Broccoli (and its cousins, cauliflower, kale and Brussels sprouts)

- Onions and garlic

- Artichokes

- Fiber such as whole grains

- Nuts/seeds

- Seaweed (hijiki, dombu, wakame

- Spices such as ginger and turmeric

- Red Berries

- Yogurt

- Citrus fruits

- Water

Green tea is an amazing antioxidant and I'm listing it separate because it has amazing health benefits. Green tea is actually one of the most healing foods available. Green tea comes from the same plant as the more-familiar black tea, but it is dried whereas black tea is fermented.
Green tea does have some caffeine but the lift that comes from a cup of green tea is less than coffee because of the amino acid *theanine*. This amino acid works to counteract the caffeine by promoting production of calming brain neurotransmitters.
You can purchase green tea in tea bags or as loose tea. When allergy symptoms appear (or cold or flu), begin to up your intake of cups of hot green tea. You are zapping your immune system with added antioxidants and calming your nervous system all at the same time.

As you can see, the lists of ways you can support and revive your immune system are many and varied. Most are simple to implement into your daily lifestyle, just a little discipline is all that is required. The dividends that are enjoyed as a result are beyond your ability to calculate.

Chapter 8
Know Your Triggers

One of the under-appreciated benefits of optimum health is that you begin to *hear* your body talking to you. You will learn to listen and understand the signals the body is giving out. One of the major problems with medication is the *masking* that happens. Medications mask over the symptoms which is like putting a piece of duct tape over your mouth; all attempts of communication are thwarted. You are reduced to a lot of hand waving, stomping of feet, or nodding of the head.

When the voice of the body is stifled, it will remain quiet for a time. But sooner or later it will have to make its needs known and the results can be quite unpleasant. In some cases, downright dangerous.

Learning about your body and how it functions is to respect your body. Listening to your body is also respect for your body. Your body may be crying out for rest, or for nutrition, or for a break from sugar overload, or for a simple drink of water. Will you hear?

In our rush through life, we take many of our bodily functions totally for granted. The old heart is still ticking, the breath is going out and in, all the limbs are taking you where you want to go and performing needed tasks. So there's no big deal, right?

But you're reading this book because there *is* a big deal. You saw the title and you were interested because you are fed up with suffering from allergies that rob you of joy, peace, and health, so you wanted to know more.

It's time to stop taking for granted that wonderful machine we call our body. It's time to give it all the care and attention it deserves.

Purchase a special notebook – one small enough to carry around with you. (Or you can set up a special file on your computer or iPad.) Begin to chart the allergic symptoms as they appear. The more you chart the triggers and the patterns, the more in tune you will be with your body. Then you can cooperate in the battle.

- When did they start? (Time of day; time of month; season; etc.)

- Where were you?

- What possible allergens were you in contact with?

- When they started were you unduly stressed?

- Were you overly tired?

- Log your nutritional intake so you can reflect back. Had you been *eating on the run grabbing whatever* and then the symptoms set in?

- What medications did you take?

- How long did you have to keep taking the medication before you got relief?

Log every detail you can think of that is in any way related to your allergic reaction. The more you log, the more you will see patterns forming. These patterns will be clues in how and why you are suffering from such severe reactions.

You may not be a detail-type personality and this may sound like a lot of busywork and drudgery to you. But just how serious are you about getting well? The more serious you are the more determined you will be to chart your course to wellness.

Think of when you first met a new friend. You wanted to get to know that person better, and so the two of you exchanged a long list of questions. The questions and answers fired back and forth as you learned more about one another. Will that be the gist of the conversation every time you get together from then on? Probably not. The initial conversation is to get to know one another.

This initial journaling is so you can get to know *you*. Your allergic reactions are trying to tell you something. It's up to you to find out what. You are the detective; you are the sleuth. Time to solve the long-standing mystery.

How long you will need to journal is up to you. The majority of allergic people who embark on this journey to optimum health report that as they incorporate discipline to change their lifestyle they experience a marked reduction in the occurrence and the severity of allergic reactions. They don't purposely stop taking medication, it just happens. They go for longer and longer periods of time symptom-free so there's no need for the inhaler, the nasal spray, that antihistamines, the allergy shots. It's an amazing transformation.

Maintain your vigilance by using your progress chart (or journal) until you experience successful results.

Conclusion

In no way is this book meant to be considered an extensive report on the condition of allergies. Rather it is written as an overview to create an awareness. An awareness for allergy sufferers that alternatives exist to the conventional treatments that treat symptoms only, but never the root cause. In Chapter 4, we looked at a number of areas in which our culture has changed over the past several decades. We know it's foolish to think we could ever go back to quieter, more peaceful times. However, there are many ways in which you can replicate some of that peace and quiet, and replicate the dietary practices that have been lost along the way.

Take time during your hurried life to rest and reflect. If there is a shady park near where you live, go there often. Connect with nature by sitting still and listening to the birds and watching the clouds. If you are a total city dweller, try to get out of that environment at least once a quarter. Find a quiet spot in the country where you can let your body and mind rest and recuperate.

Get proper rest; drink plenty of water. Exercise and deep breathe to introduce plenty of needed oxygen. Eat foods in their natural state. Wean yourself from junk foods that do nothing to nourish your body. Wean yourself from heavy sugar intake. Supply your body with all that it needs to function properly. Do this in the same way you would care for your new car by supplying all that it needs to run properly. By caring for your body you are now supporting all of the warfare systems needed to fight off the invader allergens that at one time overpowered your system. Now your healthy system will overpower and defeat the allergens. And you come out the winner.

Here's to your good health and your allergy-free life.

To work with Michael Von Irvin or make comments contact
help@writersprofitguide.com

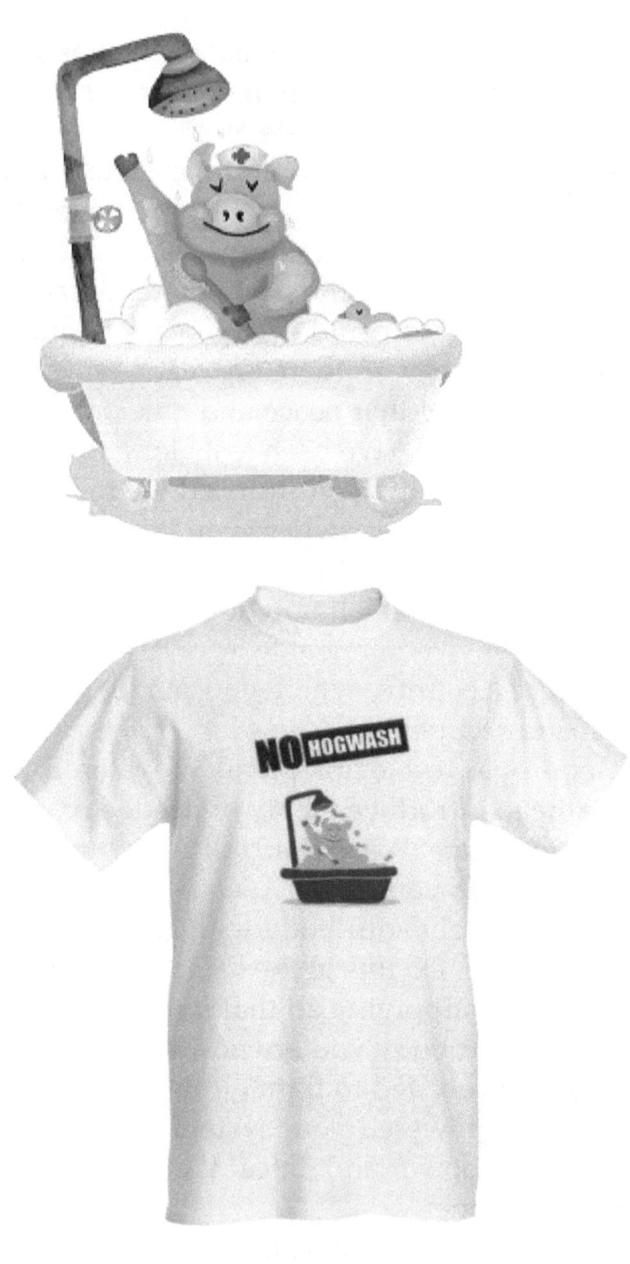

NO HOGWASH

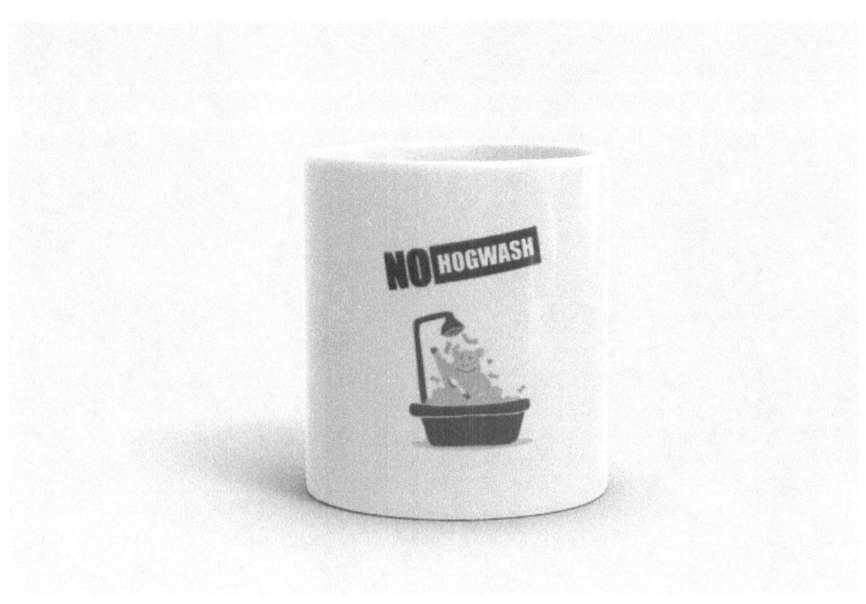

To work with Michael Von Irvin or make comments contact
help@writersprofitguide.com